Fitness For Senior Citizens With Limited Mobility

I0417287

Don't Let Your Limited Mobility Stop You From Exercising!

RON KNESS

Contents

Disclaimer

This publication is for informational purposes only and is not intended as medical advice. Medical advice should always be obtained from a qualified medical professional for any health conditions or symptoms associated with them.

Every possible effort has been made in preparing and researching this material. We make no warranties with respect to the accuracy, applicability of its contents or any omissions.

See your healthcare professional before starting any diet, health or exercise program!

The Benefits of Exercising

The benefits of exercise for your body are so much wider than most people ever imagine. Everyone knows that exercise helps you to maintain a healthy weight.

We have all been lectured on cardiovascular exercise to keep our hearts in shape. Most of us know that walking helps to increase circulation and lower blood pressure. What is surprising is the benefits of exercise for just about every other part of your life, as well – especially as you age.

One of the benefits of exercise is that it increases your lifespan. Regular exercise, along with a healthy diet, decreases your chances of dying prematurely. That is probably the best benefit of exercise and a major reason to begin an exercise program.

Working out lowers blood pressure and the risk of heart attack or stroke. It decreases the risk of many chronic diseases including diabetes. Regular walking can promote blood flow to the legs and feet, increasing healing 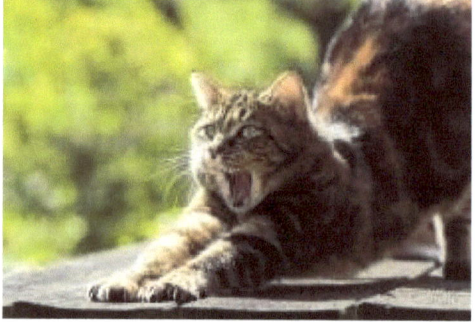 potential. Not only do people who exercise live longer lives, but they have less pain in later life.

The benefits of exercise not only benefit you physically, but also mentally. As a matter-of-fact, it is crucial for your brain health.

Being in control of your body weight and form can actually elevate your mood. Exercise decreases depression and mood swings for people with even severe forms of depression.

It also helps you by increasing your self-esteem. Regular daily exercise promotes self-discipline that spills over into the rest of your life. People who exercise regularly tend to have more social interaction than people who do not. This in turn stimulates the brain, especially in the elderly; it increases memory function and mental acuity.

Regular exercise improves your sex life. I have been told *"Men who exercise regularly are much less likely to experience erectile dysfunction or impotence than men who do not exercise."* And it makes sense.

The reason being, simple cardiovascular exercises increase blood flow to all of your organs. It helps to increase your stamina and your sexual functioning. And who couldn't use a little more time between the sheets with your loved one!

Physically, exercise decreases your risk of osteoporosis, heart attack, and stroke – it even decreases your cholesterol levels. If your doctor is preaching to you about lowering your triglycerides, exercise can help you. It is shown to prevent certain forms of cancer, including breast cancer.

Women who exercise regularly are 60% less likely to develop breast cancer than women who do not exercise. Even moderate exercise can reverse insulin dependent diabetes.

Exercises help your body gain muscle and lose fat. It creates alternate pathways for blood flow, helping to bypass clogged arteries; it lowers your heart rate, increases your lung capacity and creates a toned body that works at optimal capacity. Working out even helps you sleep better at night – important because this is when your body repairs itself.

A body's temperature lowers naturally a few hours after exercise. This helps even an insomniac get a better night's rest. And when you are awake, exercise also increases your energy levels, meaning you can accomplish more when you exercise.

With the benefits of exercise so vast, it is surprising that anyone would want to avoid working out. Unfortunately, exercise is sometimes pushed aside because we have so many other things to do with our time – seniors are busy! But one of the things you should make time to do is exercise because of the many and varied benefits derived from doing it.

4 Group Assisted Living Workouts

If you live in an assisted living facility, you benefit not only from possible on-site fitness resources, and maybe even a gym, but the fact that you can exercise with others who live there. This can help to motivate you and keep you energized, while also getting in a good workout regularly. Here are some different workouts you can do with a group at an assisted living facility.

1. Dance Class

If your assisted living community offers dance classes, you should definitely consider taking one! These can be so much fun, and because they are held at your community, all of the dance moves are going to cater to your physical capabilities. There are even seniors in wheelchairs or who can't spend a lot of time walking or standing who love taking these dance classes. Plus, it is a great way to meet your neighbors and make some really close friends.

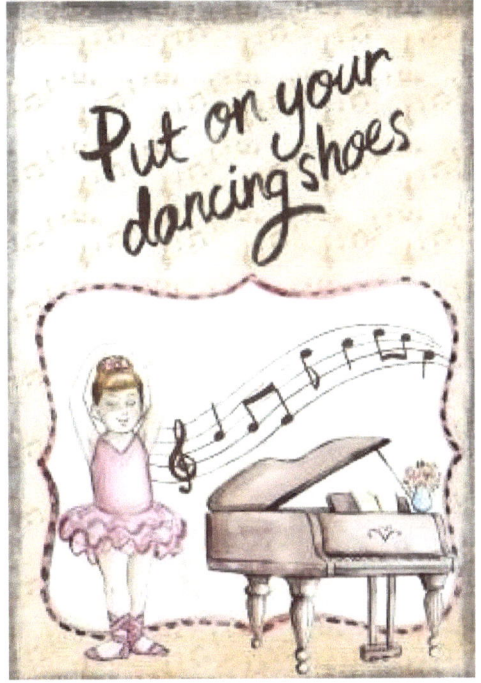

2. Aerobics

There are two types of aerobics classes that assisted living communities often provide, including regular low-impact aerobics and water aerobics. If you have a large community that has a swimming pool, then water aerobics can be great for you. This is ideal because it is gentle on your body, so even if you have bad arthritis, water exercising allows you to get in a good workout without too much stress being put on your joints.

You can also take a regular low-impact aerobics class with other seniors in your community. This will provide very simple movements to get your blood pumping without causing physical discomfort, such as walking in place, lifting your legs, and moving your arms.

3. Circuit Training

Do you have a workout room or fitness center in your assisted living facility? If so, you can take advantage of by going to a circuit training session. There are usually multiple machines in one room, where each person uses one machine for a short period of time, then moves to the next machine. You do this as a group so you get the community factor, but you also get to use different workout machines for great results.

4. Outdoor Workouts

Many assisted living communities provide different outdoor activities that allow you to also exercise, such as playing golf or tennis, going for a walk around the community, or playing games like badminton.

This is another wonderful way to make friends, socialize, and move your body at the same time.

5 Solo Assisted Living Workouts

You may live in an assisted living community with other seniors, but that doesn't mean you are interested in exercising with them. But don't worry, there are plenty of workouts you can do in the facility all by yourself! Here are some different solo assisted living workout options you might have.

1. Bed or Chair Workouts

It is good to start with these types of workouts, because you shouldn't feel like because you are in a wheelchair or bedridden, you can't still exercise. There are a lot of workouts you can still do, from gentle yoga or leg lifts in the bed, to upper body workouts if you are in a wheelchair. These can be done on your own right in your room, so it is often more comfortable as well.

2. Yoga and Stretching

These are great exercises to do on your own because they are gentle on your body and really improve your flexibility and balance, which is important as you get older. You can do them in your room, or use the facility's workout room if you have one. Make sure you are doing the more gentle and senior-friendly yoga poses like the mountain pose and tree pose.

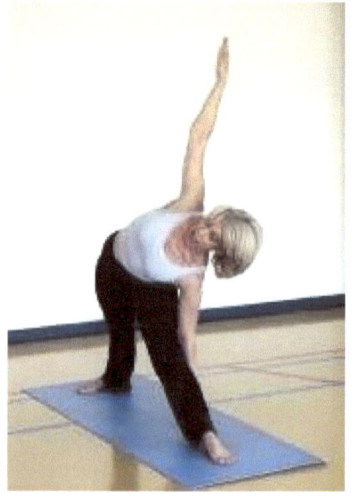

With stretching, just do different movements that feel comfortable and allow you to stretch different parts of your body.

3. Walking or Jogging

This will depend on your fitness level and what you feel comfortable with, but both walking and jogging are ideal workouts to do on your own. If you are physically fit, jogging can be a great workout for you, and you can control how far you go or how long you jog for. Walking 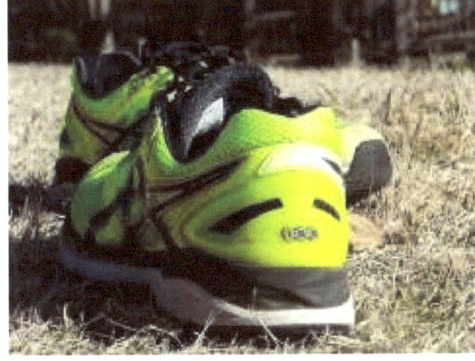 is good for most seniors, even if you only walk for 5-10 minutes a day around the assisted living community.

4. Gardening

Does your assisted living community have a garden they let everyone use? If so, this is the perfect workout! You are able to get outside and enjoy all that vitamin D, while also getting more energy from the sun. Gardening can be a rewarding activity that also provides excellent fat and calorie burning. Ask for knee pads or a chair if your body gets sore from doing the gardening.

5. In-Room Workouts

Perhaps you are someone that prefers exercising from inside your room, and that is okay. There are workout DVDs and television channels that provide easy workouts for you to do right in front of your TV.

Assisted Living Workouts Without Gym Equipment

Many assisted living facilities will have a workout room or fitness center, which is great news! You don't have to leave the facility just to use workout equipment, and you can typically use it at any time during the day based on your personal schedule.

Strength Training

The first type of workout you can do if your assisted living facility has a workout room or full gym is to use the weight training equipment. There are a lot of different types of equipment, so just use whatever is available. Perhaps they are set up 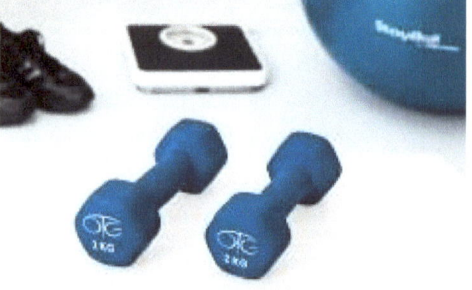 for circuit training, where multiple machines are set up in a large circle, allowing you to use each machine for a short period of time. Other workout rooms just have a single full-body workout machine, so ask someone who works there to teach you how to use this type of machine. Strength training is going to help keep your body in good shape and will also improve your flexibility and balance, two things that are important as a senior adult.

Cardio Equipment

If there is a workout room, you probably also have some cardio equipment you can use. This allows you to get your blood pumping and improve your circulation, without having to go for a long walk or take an aerobics class. Perhaps you would prefer just using a treadmill or elliptical, both machines will provide a good workout. The treadmill is good if you want to walk or jog, without going outside. You can usually set different speeds and even change the incline. With an elliptical, it provides upper and lower body workouts, which is great. Then there is the stationary bike, providing a different type of lower body workout.

Gym Accessories

Lastly, there is the option of using different types of accessories in the workout room. This is a good option when you want to switch up your workout routine, or when the heavy equipment is a little hard on your joints. For 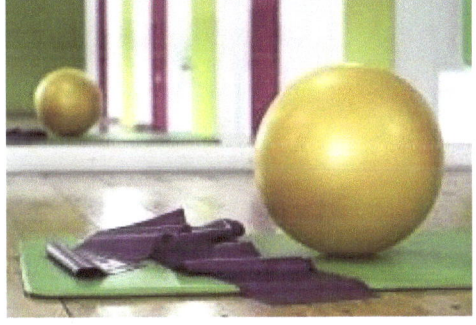 example, resistance bands are often easier to handle than some of the other weightlifting equipment, but just as effective. To work on your balance, you can use a medicine ball for some workouts. If you prefer, there are usually hand weights in fitness centers or workout rooms, allowing you to choose a lighter weight that is easier for you to handle.

Exercises For Seniors With Arthritis

Arthritis is a painful condition that causes your joints to be inflamed and sore, and is hard to deal with, let alone get in exercise. However, moving your body is important when you have arthritis. The following exercises are gentle enough for you to do even if you suffer from arthritis.

Chair Stand

If you have severe arthritis pain, you probably struggle with standing or walking for long periods of time. That is what makes the chair stand exercise so perfect. It gets your body moving and allows you to stand up, which is important with this condition, but it won't cause too much discomfort for you. You should use a chair that is comfortable and keeps your body upright, but isn't hard to get out of. Avoid using a recliner or couch when doing the chair stand. To do this exercise, you will simply sit up in the chair, stand up off the chair, then sit back down. This works on your leg muscles and can also help with balance.

Water Walking

You are in luck if your assisted living community has a swimming pool, or if you can go to a gym that has one. Not only are there water aerobics classes, but water walking exercises are excellent when you have arthritis.

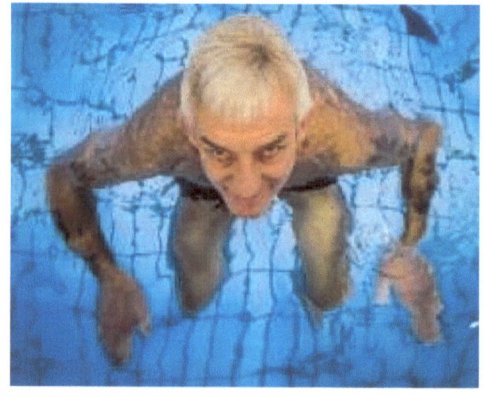

All you need to do is stand in the shallow end of the pool and start walking in place or trying to move a little bit while walking under the water. This gets your body moving, but it isn't too hard on your legs and other joints that might be hurting you.

Yoga

You are going to see a lot of recommendations for yoga, and that is because it is ideal for seniors, especially those living in an assisted living community. Yoga is very versatile, allowing you to modify most of the movements, take your time to learn, and get tons of health benefits. You can do it with or without a working DVD, on your own in your room, outside, or in a class with others in the community.

The important thing when it comes to yoga is that you don't push yourself too hard and try to do moves that are uncomfortable for you. Yoga should not be painful or cause you to wake up and be sore. Do gentle, easy movements and only go to the more advanced ones when you have lots of practice and feel comfortable doing so.

No-Equipment Assisted Living Workouts

If you live in an assisted living community that doesn't offer exercise classes or a workout room, that's totally fine. There are plenty of workouts you can do on your own or with friends in the facility that don't use any equipment whatsoever.

Walking

This is probably the best no-equipment workout you can do when you are living in an assisted living, but also for seniors who are living in their own home. The great thing about walking is that it doesn't require much in order to do it. You can walk anywhere as long as it is safe to do, whether you walk around your assisted living community or walk down the street. If you want more of a scenic area, you can get transportation to a local beach or park and walk there. This is also something you can do alone or with others.

Dancing

It is easy to find workouts to do so that you stay in shape, but they aren't always enjoyable. If you find workout classes to be no fun for you, then why not do some dancing? This is also something just about everyone can handle. You can turn on your favorite music and dance in your room at the assisted living facility, whether alone or with others. Even if you are chair-bound, there are upper body dance moves you can do that will get you moving and help with strengthening your heart.

Stair Stepping

You probably have some types of steps or stairs at your living community, which also provides a good workout for you. All you need to do is either walk up and down all of the stairs, or just the first couple of steps. You want to pay attention to your body and not overdo it. If you have arthritis, be careful with this and just use one short step at a time. However, this provides a good, easy workout for you. Go slow and stop if you start experiencing body discomfort or pain.

Take a Workout Class

There are plenty of workout classes to consider that won't require any equipment. These are often provided right at the community, such as low-impact aerobics or yoga. Classes are great because it gets you out of your room and allows you to socialize with other seniors that you live with. Check a local community center if your assisted living facility doesn't offer exercise classes.

Seated Workouts For Seniors

Whether you have trouble standing and walking, or you are wheelchair-bound, you might be looking for ways to get your blood pumping and body moving while you are in the chair. Luckily, there are a lot of great options. Take a look at these different seated workouts you can do right in your assisted living room.

Seated Toe Taps

If you are in a wheelchair or need to sit on a chair, but you

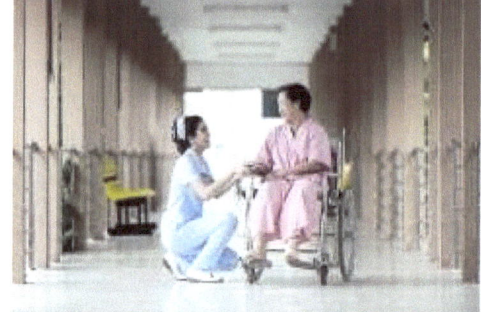

still have movement in your legs, then you can try toe taps. These will help to work on the strength in your legs, while getting your body moving in the chair. All you need to do is sit in your chair and keep your heels flat on the ground. Take just your toes and bend them up, then tap them back down by touching the ground. It can be helpful if you are able to move toward the front edge of the chair, but if you are in a wheelchair, you definitely don't need to do this. Try to hold the toes up for a few seconds each time, and do about 10 repetitions for each foot.

Knee Lifts

Another exercise you can try if you have movement of your lower body is knee lifts. Be aware that this also works your abdominal muscles, so if you recently had surgery in your abdomen area, you might want to skip this one for now.

However, if you are fine in the legs and abdomen, give it a try. The knee lifts are simply done by sitting in your chair and lifting one of your knees up and as close to your chest as you can get it. Hold for a few seconds, put it down, then try it with the other leg. Go for about 10 on each side.

Chair Aerobics

Yes, there is aerobics for those who are seated! Chair aerobics basically is a type of low-impact aerobics that allows you to move your arms and legs as much as possible, burn calories, and get your blood pumping through your body. If you don't have movement in the lower part of your body, you can just do the upper body chair aerobics exercises.

Balance Exercises

Lastly, there are some seated balance exercises that are going to work on your strength and flexibility. One of them is a sit to stand movement, so this does require standing, but not for a long time. Then there are others where you don't leave the chair, like hip extensions, side leg raises, knee raises, leg lifts, and various arm exercises.

Stretching and Balance Exercises For Seniors

While many seniors focus a lot on walking or using the fitness room in their assisted living facility, not many consider the importance of stretching and balance exercises. These are going to support your body as you age, making just about everything a little easier for you. If the facility where you live doesn't provide stretching classes, you can still do these exercises in the comfort of your own room.

Tips For Flexibility Movements

Before you learn about the different balance and stretching

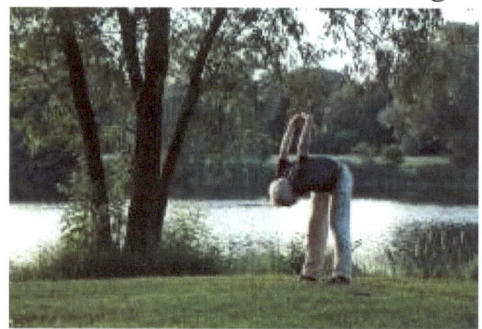

exercises that will help with your flexibility and overall balance, you need to follow these guidelines. They act as safety precautions to help you avoid injury or major soreness after performing the movements. First of all, you always want to warm up before doing any type of exercise, from walking to doing yoga for balance. Also make sure during each stretch, you are not bouncing; this can happen if you are extending the joint too far. Slowly extend the joint to the point where it starts to feel tight, then stop and hold it there for 15 to 20 seconds. Then slowly retract back to the fully relaxed position.

During stretches, you should not be holding your breath, so make sure you exhale on the stretch and inhale on the return! Also be gentle when stretching, as these exercises are not meant to cause pain. Be gentle with your body.

Hippie Stretch

This first stretching movement is going to work on your flexibility and balance. The hippie stretch is done while standing with your feet together. Keep your feet flat on the ground, then bend forward and start walking your hands down your legs. Only go as far as you can while it still feels comfortable. Your head should dangle down while holding the stretch for about 10-15 seconds. Slowly work your hands back up to the starting position. Go up and down a few times while performing this stretch.

Overhead Stretch

Another stretch that can be really good for you is going to work on your triceps, helping to stretch out your arms. Since you are standing while performing this exercise, it also helps work on your balance at the same time. You want to stand with your feet apart, making sure your shoulders are back. Reach one arm up pointing the ceiling, then bend at the elbow and let your hand fall behind your back to stretch it out. Hold this for a few seconds, then alternative to the other arm. You can do a few repetitions of this stretch.

Keep in mind doing gentle yoga poses also provide some exceptional stretching, balance, and flexibility exercises for you. We talk about some simple ones in the next chapter.

Simple Yoga Poses for Seniors

Yoga is an excellent workout to do if you are a senior and living in an assisted living community. Many of these communities offer yoga classes, adjusting the moves for your mobility level. However, you can also do yoga in your own room if you prefer the privacy with these types of moves.

Mountain Pose

The mountain pose is a simple and gentle yoga pose that

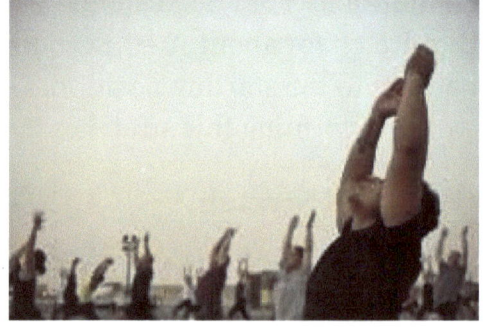

works on your balance, while also not being too difficult. Not only is it good for seniors, but this pose is good for anyone who is new to doing yoga. This is a standing pose where your feet are together and touching. You want to tighten your abdominal muscles and relax your shoulders. Take a few deep breaths, reaching your arms up, forming the mountain pose. If you have difficulty with your posture, this yoga pose can help with that.

Downward Facing Dog

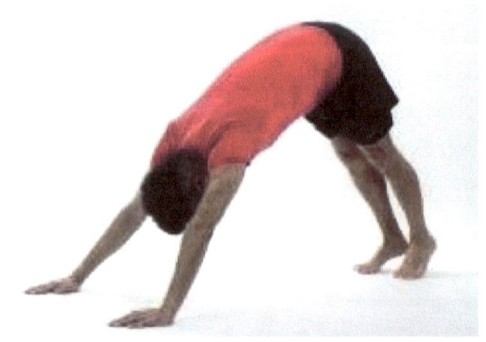

This is a very common yoga pose many people like to perform, which can also be done as a senior adult.

20

It is ideal for improving your strength and flexibility. However, if you have pain in your wrists, you will need to do a modification called the forearm downward dog. This is a pose done on the floor, where you are on your hands and knees, then move your body up so your bottom is in the air and you are performing a triangle motion. If you have wrist pain, hold your body up on your forearms instead of your hands.

You can also go to a senior yoga class, which shows you moves that are gentle for your body, but also some modifications if you need them. If you want, you can also get some others in the community together and do these types of yoga poses outdoors. You get fresh air and it can be fun switching to a new environment.

Tree Pose

Another standing yoga pose that is good for seniors to do either alone or in a group is the tree pose. This is a standing pose, so it also helps with your balance and strength, similar to the mountain pose. Like the mountain pose, your legs should be together with your big toes touching during the initial stage of the tree pose.

Now, reach your arms over your head and keep your palms together. Raise one leg a little off the ground, holding it for 10-15 seconds, then releasing. Repeat this with the other leg.

Try These Workouts In Bed

When you are living in an assisted living facility, it is not always possible to get up and go to the workout room or even go for a walk. On days when you are bedridden, such as following an illness or procedure, you should still try to move your body as much as possible. These workouts are going to help you do that.

Leg Lifts

If you are bedridden, it is really important that you move as much of your body as you can. Unless you just had surgery on your legs, ankles, or feet, you should try some leg lifts. This will get your circulation going and at least give you some movement until you are able to get out of bed. Plus, leg lifts not only work on your leg muscles, but can also engage your abs and lower back as well. You can lift your legs one at a time either bent or straight while lying on your back, or you can do side leg lifts when laying on your side. These are simple exercises you can do while watching TV, so it really is a good way to keep moving while you are in bed.

Palm Stretch

The next exercise can be done in bed and is something you can do even after surgery or with a severe illness. The palm stretch is going to help to stretch out and move your hands, wrists, and arms, which also improves your circulation. Gradually moving and stretching different body parts is vital to handling bed rest and possibly one day getting out of bed without too much pain or immobility.

A palm stretch is done by opening your palm and stretching out your fingers, then trying to touch your palm with each finger, one at a time. That is all that is needed.

Bed Yoga

Yoga is a recommended exercise for seniors in an assisted living facility, because it is something you can do alone or in a group, and many communities even offer classes. However, you can also do it right in your own bed with some simple moves. There is the happy baby pose, which might have a silly name, but can be effective. You just lay on your back and bend your knees, then hold onto your feet as you do so. Try to hold it for 5-10 breaths. If you can handle it, pulling your knees to your chest and holding it is another good yoga pose to do in bed.

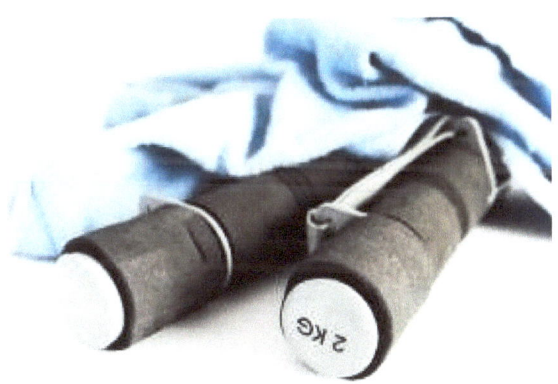

Why Every Senior Should Be Walking

One of the best exercises for seniors to do is walking. Many doctors will recommend this for seniors as long as they are not wheelchair-bound, because it provides so many different health benefits and is something pretty much anyone can do. Here are some things to know about walking as it relates to seniors, particularly those living in assisted living facilities.

It is Good For Your Joints

If you have arthritis, or soreness in your joints, then walking might just be the best activity for you. Walking can be easy on your joints when you choose the right walking surface, plus it helps to get your body moving, which is important when you have arthritis. Walking also helps to support your joints, because the movement allows the fluid in the joints to circulate properly. If you have a lot of pain, just walk for 5-10 minutes to start with, gradually increasing the time as you feel more comfortable.

You Have Full Control Over the Workout

Something to keep in mind when it comes to walking is that you have full control over the workout. You can decide how long you want to walk, choose different locations, and even control the speed and intensity. It helps you to customize the workout according to your fitness and comfort level.

Walking Helps With Circulation

Walking is also really great for your circulation, which is super important as a senior adult. As you begin to age, your risk for heart disease and high blood pressure increases gradually. It is important to do everything you can to lower your risk, which also includes improving your circulation. If you are sitting for long periods of time without moving your body, it can do quite a bit of damage to your circulation. Just take a short walk each day can really help with your circulation, plus providing all of the other amazing health benefits.

It Can Help to Lower Your Blood Sugar

This is one of the reasons you should try taking at least a short walk every day after you have eaten your dinner. Your blood sure might be a little elevated after eating dinner, especially if you have diabetes or are even borderline diabetes. With a short walk of at least 10-15 minutes after dinner, you are able to lower your blood sugar, which is good news if you do have diabetes. There is a blood sugar spike usually for a few hours after a big meal, so keep this in mind when deciding when you want to walk each day.

Final Thoughts

If you exercise, the idea that you'll live longer is a guarantee. But getting out of bed for that workout isn't as easy as you'd like it to be. It's cold in the winter, dark outside and who wants to hit the pavement jogging at the hour?

Or finishing up work when your body is zapped of all its strength and you think you can't possibly do more than fire up the television at home, let alone hit the gym, can be a real trial.

Yet, just like an apple a day keeps the doctor away, you know that exercise does so much good for your body. If only exercise weren't so hard to get around to doing! You know what's said about exercise. You've heard it all.

Exercising gives you more body strength, raises your stamina, helps fight against heart attacks, keeps your blood pressure at a good level and even gives you more self-esteem. You might even know that starting a regular exercise routine right now will make it easier on your body to get around when you're older.

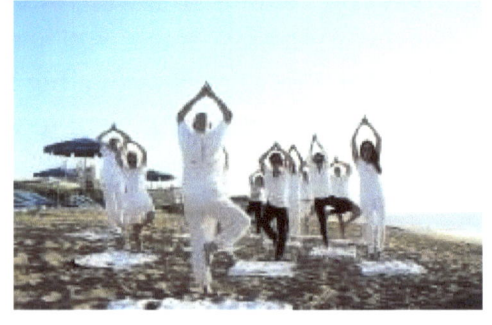

But it's still hard for you to find the motivation to move. Here are some ways that you can make exercise a part of your life and even learn to love it.

If you don't focus on the hard work of exercise, living longer won't just be a wish, but a more concrete possibility.

Who doesn't want to be around long enough to do what they've always wanted to do? See the world? Be active with your grandchildren or significant other? Celebrate an eightieth birthday? Or hundredth?

While it's true that exercise tones the muscles so that you look healthy and fit on the outside, exercise gets those organs healthy and fit on the inside of the body, too. Every organ in the body can stay healthier longer with exercise.

When you exercise, the kidney functions are improved as you tone your body and get rid of any unnecessary fat. When you carry the best amount of weight for your body's framework, you make the job your organs have to do a lot easier and they don't have to work as hard.

Exercising can boost your lung function, keep your heart beating at maximum potential and can help joint pain that's caused by arthritis. The worst thing you can do for your body is to sit around and not exercise. You subtract time from your life. Time you could give to yourself and your loved ones.

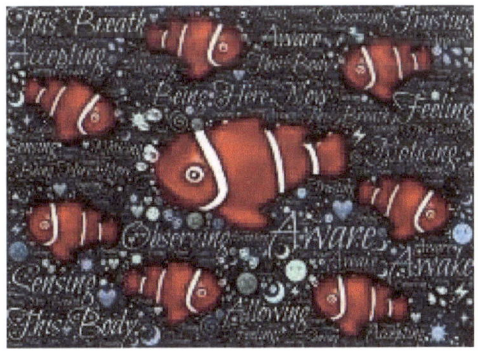

So how do you exercise, live longer, if you absolutely dread it? You learn to reward yourself. Use a chart if you need to and for each half an hour that you exercise, give yourself a treat.

It could be something as simple as buying yourself a new outfit, picking up an item for your home or putting aside money for a big ticket item. Reward yourself when you reach certain milestones.

Exercised a week without fail? Or went a month and stuck to the routine? Then you should treat yourself. Set both short term and long term goals. Not only will your body get rewarded by feeling better, but you'll find that you're looking forward the rewards you give yourself. For a long term goal, you might try the reward of taking a vacation somewhere you've always wanted to go.

Other Relevant Books by This Author

If you would like to read more relevant books about this topic, here is a list of the CreateSpace links, titles and descriptions from this author:

https://www.createspace.com/6107842

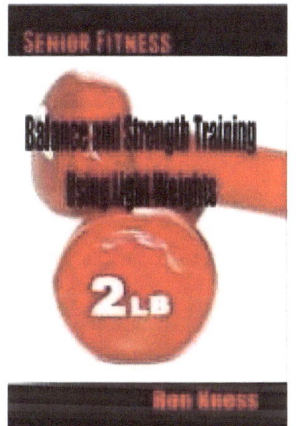

Senior Fitness - Balance and Strength Training Using Light Weights

As you age you notice that you are not as strong as before. Most of us simply chalk that up to the "natural" aging process. However, to fight the physical dangers of aging, strength is very important.

We are not talking about bodybuilding and packing on bulky muscles. What we mean is simply making your body stronger so that you don't become part of one of the following statistics ...

• Falls in those 75 or older contribute to 70% of accidental deaths.
• Respiratory issues such as COPD are the #3 cause of death for men and women 65 and older.
• 1 in every 3 people over 65 will fall each year. (Doctors are certain this number is drastically higher, since many falls are not reported because of embarrassment or concern over medical bills.)
• 1 in 5 Americans over 65 suffer from a lack of independence and reduced quality of life due to osteoporosis and/or diabetes.

• If you are 80 years or older, there is a 50% chance you will fall.

• As a senior citizen, if you fall once, you are 200% to 300% more likely to fall again.

• Heart disease impacts 26% of women and 37% of men 65 or older.

 • Roughly 9,500 deaths in older US citizens each year are associated with falling.

 • Even if you survive a fall as a senior citizen, you suffer a much greater functional decline in your ability to perform normal daily activities.

 • Over 250,000 older Americans experience a fractured hip each year (research as of 1996, probably a larger number now due to aging of the US population)

• Over half of adults over 65 years of age are affected by arthritis.

• 1 in 4 seniors who fracture a hip die within 6 months as a result of that injury.

The real problem here is not the scary statistics just covered. The problem is that each and every one of the debilitating and even deadly issues we just mentioned can be positively impacted by simply lifting light weights, yet seniors are not strength training.

The following are the incredible benefits of simply lifting light weights a few times each week for seniors ...

• A feeling of self-esteem and self-confidence
• Improved circulatory system
• Lowered risk of heart disease
• Regulation of a naturally healthy body weight
• Light weightlifting is an effective way to treat and eradicate back pain
• You have fewer feelings of depression, anxiety and stress
• You strengthen your bones, naturally improving your ability to fight health issues like osteoporosis

• Light weightlifting is excellent for preventing and treating diabetes
• Arthritis sufferers experience fewer painful symptoms when they weight train regularly
• Your balance and flexibility are boosted, and joint pain is reduced.

By now you are probably sold on the fact that you need to be lifting light weights and strength training if you are over 50 years of age or older.

So, what's your next step?

Reserve your copy of this book that shows you exactly how to benefit from lifting light weights as a senior citizen.

https://www.createspace.com/6096479

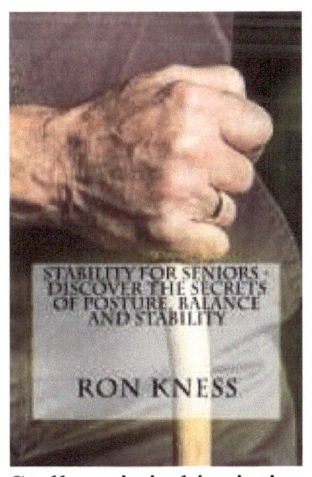

Stability for Seniors - Discover the Secrets of Posture, Balance and Stability

You may have noticed that some people in your neighborhood, who are in their 60s, have trouble walking and getting around. Yet, if you look at Sylvester Stallone, he is still muscular and in excellent shape. He is still directing and getting physical in his action movies.

Stallone is in his sixties.

What about Arnold Schwarzenegger? His arms and muscles are bigger than those of men half his age.

He doesn't seem to lack coordination or balance.

The dancer, Michael Flatley, is 57 and still dancing. The former model, Christie Brinkley, is sixty and she is as elegant and fit as ever.

What is the underlying reason here? Why these people are healthy and well-coordinated while you or others you may know are sickly, unfit or unable to move without assistance?

The answer is – the life choices we made.

Many people sacrifice their health in pursuit of their career. They are so busy making a living that they neglect to make a life. The excuse that they do not have time to exercise is tossed about so frequently that they end up letting their health and fitness slide.

If you are not regularly active, you will have muscular atrophy over time. Your flexibility will decrease. Your core strength will diminish. As time progresses, you will be less limber and more rigid.

This is exactly how people age poorly. It's a process that has snowballed over time.

Only with regular exercise and a healthy diet can you have a body that is fit and has the ability to almost reverse aging.

If you have neglected your health for years and life seems to be a chore now because you can't get around without assistance, do not feel dejected.

You can remedy the situation. You can restore the strength, balance and stamina that you have lost.

It is never too late to become what you might have been.

Your body will help you, if you help it.

This guide will show you exactly what you need to do to restore your balance, strengthen your core and give you the ability to live life to its fullest. Read how …

https://www.createspace.com/6328327

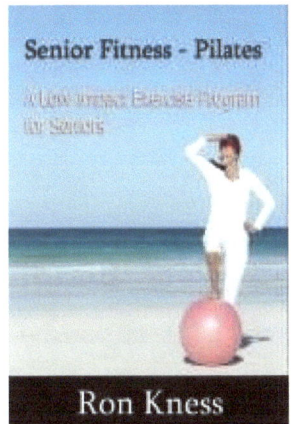

Senior Fitness: Pilates: The Low Impact Exercise Program for Seniors

Do you wake up in the morning feeling lethargic? Do you wish you had the energy to run around with kids once again? Feel stiff and aching bones?

If you answered yes to any 1 of those 3 questions, then pay attention because what you are about to read in the next few minutes could change your life

Firstly, What exactly is the problem? Generally it is inactivity. Studies have shown that it only takes a few days of lying in bed to start losing your strength, flexibility and balance.

Once this happens you are at risk of beginning the dreaded downward health spiral. If you are looking to take care of your body and remain youthful well into your twilight years then it's important to not let anything stand in your way from doing it. Don't let a few dollars stop you from learning the secrets that could change your life while also enriching it.

Here are just some of the things you'll learn in this book:

==> Chapter 1 – Discover How Activity Promotes Longevity.
==> Chapter 2 - The History of Pilates
==> Chapter 3 - What exactly is Pilates? Should I be doing it?
==> Chapter 4 - The Benefits of Pilates
==> Chapter 5 - Steps Before Beginning Pilates
==> Chapter 6 - What to Expect in a First Session.
==> Chapter 7 – 4 Fantastic Pilates Moves To Do.
==> Chapter 8 - Avoiding Common Pitfalls
==> Chapter - Making Exercise/Pilates Part of Lifestyle
==> Advanced Chapter – Taking Things Up a Notch

Get your copy today before it is too late!

About the Author

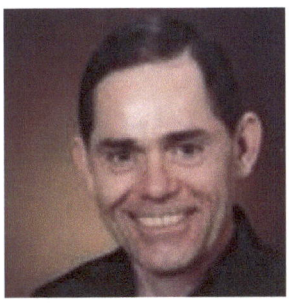

I have published over 125 books on Amazon for Kindle, CreateSpace and other publishing platforms.

While most of my books are on health and fitness in general, as I age (now 65) at the time of this writing) my topics of interest are geared toward aging baby boomers and older.

Besides my own writing, I also ghostwrite ebooks, books, reports, articles, blogs and do Kindle conversions for clients on a variety of topics.

Today my wife and I are retired from our careers and live in Gold Canyon, AZ. I now write as a retirement business where you'll find me happily sitting in my office typing away on my laptop as I work on my next book or ghostwriting project . . . that is if we are not traveling on a cruise ship - our new-found mode of travel.

www.ingramcontent.com/pod-product-compliance
Lightning Source LLC
Chambersburg PA
CBHW050851290526
45792CB00002B/607